Easy Juicing Recipes

Athletes Energy Drink To Improve Your
Energy And Increase Your Performance

Table of Contents

Introduction

Chapter 1: What Should Be In A Sports Drink?

Chapter 2: Natural Sports Drinks

Chapter 3: Juices vs. Smoothies

Chapter 4: Juicing Recipes for Athletes

Chapter 5: Juice Recipes To Fight Inflammation

Essential Nutrients And Minerals For Faster Recovery
1. Branched-Chain Amino Acids (BCAAS)
2. Carbohydrates
3. Antioxidants
4. Creatine Monohydrate
5. Electrolytes
Juicing Tips
5 Juicing Recipes To Help Your Body Recover Faster

Chapter 1: What Should Be In A Sports Drink?

The right sports energy drink should be rich in carbohydrates, which is obviously the most efficient source of energy. It should also contain electrolytes that are lost along with body fluid as we sweat. Electrolytes are positive ions in our bodies that are charged for electrical conduction. They are from minerals like sodium, magnesium, calcium, and potassium. The main reason electrolytes are important in an athlete's body is that they are responsible for maintaining the right PH levels. Correct PH levels create electrical impulse balance that promotes muscle cell functions during exercise.

Normally, sweat rates will differ. You may be the athlete who loses 1 kg of water heavily concentrated with high levels of sodium or one who loses 3kgs of water but with very little potassium or sodium. What matters is replacement of these electrolytes to promote rehydration for the purposes of delaying the onset of fatigue during exercise.

Types Of Sport Drinks

Sports drinks vary depending on the levels of carbohydrates, electrolytes, and fluid in them. Nevertheless, there are three kinds of sports drinks: *hypotonic, hypertonic*, and *isotonic* sports drink.

Hypotonic drinks contain a lower concentration of salt and sugar than our bodies. They quickly replace the fluid you may have lost through sweating. This type of drink is suitable for athletes who need fluid without a boost of their carbohydrate levels.

Hypertonic drinks contain a higher concentration of sugar and salt than what is in our bodies. This kind of drink works best when consumed after a work out to supplement the daily carbohydrate intake and top-up glycogen stores in the muscles. You can also use it during a long distance event to meet the high-energy demands alongside an isotonic energy drink to replace lost fluid.

Isotonic drinks have the same levels of salt and sugar as our body. The work of these drinks is to replace the fluids we lose through sweating and to boost our carbohydrate levels. This drink is most suitable for middle and long distance runners.

Chapter 2: Natural Sports Drinks

The sports drink market has many confusing and often conflicting brands; as such, it is hard to tell which ones are the best for you as an athlete. Obviously, pure clean water is the best.

Our bodies are 70% water and we lose a lot of it when we work out. It is therefore a rule of thumb that we drink at least 8 glasses of water on a normal day and more when in the field. Water helps transport oxygen and glucose throughout the body, helps maintain flexibility, and strengthens your muscles while at the same time lubricating your joints.

Failure to drink enough water could cause headaches and decreases in energy, which are all warning signs of dehydration. The problem is that after a while, plain water can get boring and it does not contain high levels of the electrolytes you lose as you exercise; hence the need to make your own natural energy drink.

Before stopping by the store to buy Gatorade on your way to the game, try making your own natural version of an energy drink: it is a lot healthier, easier, and just as fast. Why should you try making your own rather than reach for your regular store energy drinks?

Apart from the carbohydrates and electrolytes, regular sports drinks contain additional ingredients like monopotassium phosphate, natural flavors, and unnecessary artificial dyes. Some caffeinated drinks may also contain banned substances such as ephedrine, which might end up costing you your career as an athlete. A natural sports drink is a simple way out of all this.

Going natural means replacing store-bought energy drinks with juice made from fruits and vegetables. Because of their ability to improve endurance and performance, a number of major players hold some plants in high regard.

Here, we are talking about **celery**, **cucumbers**, **coconut water**, and **watermelons**. Any natural drink you juice should have at least one of them. Let us learn why each of these vegetables is important.

Celery

First, celery hydrates the body and helps keep the colon walls hydrated too. This helps get rid of hemorrhoids, a common problem you are likely to face when you are dehydrated and your diet lacks enough fiber.

Celery is also rich in electrolytes, mainly sodium and potassium. These two electrolytes combine with other electrolyte minerals in your body to provide your body with the necessary salt-ion balance that penetrates the cells and hydrates them. These two electrolytes present in celery make it ideal as the most complete fluid replacement drink.

It is important to note that sodium from common table salt or sodium chloride will not be as helpful in hydrating you. Instead, it causes bloating that upsets the stomach since it does not break down efficiently. As a result, your body sends a trigger to dump what is in the stomach. Your body perceives this as some sort of gastro intestinal threat and shuts your legs, ending your performance.

In addition to the sodium and potassium, celery also contains secondary minerals that serve the purpose of increasing your endurance. The calcium and magnesium in celery allows your muscles to continue the electrical impulse without fail even after their depletion. The main cause of cramping during and after a competition is lack of enough calcium and magnesium that are always responsible for expansion and retraction of the muscles.

When lactic acid piles up in your body, it becomes the number one limiting factor to performance. Another remarkable importance of drinking celery juice is that because of its diuretic effect, which it gets from sodium and potassium, it helps flush out these acids.

Cucumber

Many benefits in celery parallel cucumber's thus making it a great source of endurance too. Cucumbers have a water content of 96% and the nutrients in the juice cause a cooling effect in the body. This is important since the heat you produce affects your endurance as an athlete. By drinking cucumber juice, you bring down your overall body temperature, which extends your performance.

Cucumbers are also a great source of magnesium and potassium. Cucumber also has a diuretic effect that will help get rid of excess fluid in the body. Further, since the juice is alkaline in nature, it naturally helps generate energy.

The other importance of cucumber juice is that it is a great source of silica, which is a building block for your body. Your ligaments, bones, muscles, and other connective tissues use silica as a major rebuilding and repair component. Cucumber is also rich in copper, primarily responsible for moving energy around the body.

In addition, because of the other minerals it has like molybdenum, sulfur, folate, vitamin A and vitamin C, cucumber makes it possible for your body to assimilate and boost endurance.

Coconut Water

Reasons why you should add coconut water to your hydration drink are many.

First, coconut water is the most pure form of water that does not need any further distilling probably because its purification started from the ground to 30-40ft high. It is practically impossible to find any other liquid on the planet that has gone through the purification level coconut water goes through. Its purity is also because of the hard coconut shell that protects it from external elements.

Secondly, coconut water is rich in potassium; potassium boosts endurance. This electrolyte (potassium) travels to every cells in your body and is responsible for every electrical impulse for nerve conduction, the contraction of your heart, as well as skeletal muscle contraction.

Coconut water also has sodium. Sodium works to regulate the fluid in your body. Because it prevents body dehydration, it also helps flush out toxins and excess fluids. 14 ounces of coconut water contains approximately 192 mg of sodium compared to the 52 mg in Gatorade.

Because of its alkaline nature, coconut water falls in the isotonic drink category. This alkalinity makes it possible to neutralize and flash out the lactic acid in the cells and the muscles during exercise. Coconut water also contains phosphorous, an electrolyte that transfers energy throughout your body. Coconut water also has the ability to regulate your body temperature, which promotes competing for a long time without overheating.

Watermelon

Just like celery, coconut water, and cucumber, watermelon contains more than 90% water alongside the five major electrolytes. To be exact, watermelon contains 92% water, which makes it a mild diuretic. It is also rich in antioxidants like beta-carotene and lycopene that help the body protect itself from attack from sunlight, bacteria, and fungi.

Free radicals, if unchecked, can wreak havoc on your good health. For instance, they can oxidize cholesterol thus allowing it to stick to your arterial wall consequently causing strokes and heart attacks. Increased inflammation in the body, which causes rheumatoid arthritis and osteoarthritis, can also be a result of the free radicals.

The Lycopene in watermelon neutralizes these free radicals before they can start a negative chain reaction in your body. This is important to you as an athlete since your bone and joint health need to be in check for your endurance and output.

Watermelon is also rich in L-citrulline. This nutrient has an intense therapeutic effect on your muscles. Further, it extends the production of nitric oxide because the l-Arginine is recycled, which is the pre-cursor to nitric oxide.

L-citrulline also protects the l-arginine production by neutralizing the amino acid L-Arginase in the blood that destroys it. Drinking watermelon juice will give the body a more direct pathway to utilize the nitric oxide, which will boost your performance for a much longer period.

If you race in long distance marathons, bike race, or participate in ultra-endurance events, watermelon juice will keep you hydrated and deliver the essential nutrients your muscles need to maintain peak performance.

Chapter 3: Juices vs. Smoothies

Many of us tend to use these names interchangeably but freshly extracted juices are not the same as smoothies. To make smoothies, you blend fresh fruits to produce a delicious drink. This is different from extracted juice because a smoothie contains all the fiber present in the fruit.

When you place the same fruit in a juice extractor, you will end up separating the juice from the fiber. This is beneficial because you will get more nutrients from the juice without overworking your system with all that fiber. It also takes less time for the body to absorb the nutrients and your digestive system requires less energy to do so as compared to when you take the whole fruit.

Do not forget that fiber should be part of your diet so that your digestive system functions. Therefore, juices should not replace your fiber diet; rather, let the juices be an addition to a high fiber diet so that you can benefit from both.

Although fruit juices have many of the benefits mentioned above, making them green by adding vegetables would be an added advantage. Greens have a high chlorophyll content that will help oxygenate your blood. They are also rich in calcium, magnesium, and iron which are essential for your endurance. Greens also have low sugar content hence least impact in terms of blood sugar spikes.

Chapter 4: Juicing Recipes for Athletes

When selecting a juicer, choose a model that has a good quality motor (preferably 750 watts or more), one that is easy to clean, and is efficient at extracting juices from fruits, vegetables, and other leafy greens.

If you do not have a juicer, you can still use a powerful high-speed blender to blend your ingredients, and then use a fine mesh sieve to separate the liquid from chunks of veggies and all the fibers. Alternatively, you can get a big drawstring bag where you put all the pulp in there and squeeze your juice out.

If you are looking for a pre-workout energy drink or one you will drink during or after your game, the following healthy juice recipes have you covered. Enjoy!

Watermelon Cucumber Juice

Yield: 4 cups

Ingredients

4 organic lemon cucumbers or 1 large cucumber

4 cups of organic watermelon

Instructions

Cut the watermelon in half and using a spoon, scoop out chunks of its flesh to fill 4 measuring cups.

Cut the cucumbers into pieces, and then juice the cucumbers then the watermelon.

Serve immediately as is or with some ice.

Before The Gym Energy Drink

Yield: 1 serving

This drink contains Rhodiola as one of its ingredients. Rhodiola improves endurance during exercise while the combination of fructose from the berries and glucose will provide both short-term and long-term energy release.

Ingredients

1 cup of frozen berries

1 scoop of whey protein

1 tablespoon of glucose

1g of Rhodiola extract

500ml of filtered water

Instructions

Juice the berries and pour the resultant juice into a glass. Add in the other ingredients, stir, and enjoy.

Natural Electrolyte Drink

Yield: 4 servings

This drink is a great way to rehydrate after exercise. Unlike other store-bought drinks, this one does not have tons of sugar.

Ingredients

¼ cup of pineapple juice

2 tablespoons of sweetener

1 teaspoon of calcium magnesium powder

1/4 teaspoon of sea salt

1 quart of coconut water

Instructions

Slightly warm your coconut water, and then add sea salt and calcium to the mix.

Add sweetener, juice, and then mix.

Refrigerate until when ready to drink.

Energy Drink

Yield: 1 serving

This drink is full of proteins and vitamins that will give you the long lasting energy boost you will need during your performance.

Ingredients

6 oz. of very light vanilla yogurt

1 tablespoon of honey

¾ cups of light coconut milk

1 medium orange, peeled and cut

Instructions

Put the orange into your juicer and juice. Pour the juice into a glass, add the other ingredients, stir, and enjoy.

Beetroot Juice

Yield: 1 serving

The nitrate in the beets will open up your blood vessels, easing the transportation of oxygen to your muscles through the free flow of blood. Combining the beets with vegetables improves its taste and allows you to take a wider range of vitamins and nutrients.

Ingredients

1 clove of garlic

1 lemon with its rind

1 inch of ginger

2 kale leaves

3 carrots

1 fresh beet

Instructions

Juice all the ingredients and serve immediately to ensure you get the most nutrition.

High Protein Energy Drink

Yield: 2 servings

This drink is especially necessary if you are an athlete looking to build your muscles. In addition to lean meat, pineapples and kale make a great source of proteins alongside other healthy nutrients.

Ingredients

10 leaves of kale

1 big handful of parsley

1 inch-long knob of ginger

4 celery stalks

4 carrots

3 apples

1 pineapple

Instructions

Juice all the ingredients and enjoy.

Rocket Fuel Juice

Yield: 2 servings

This drink will help you feel less pain in your muscles even after a rigorous exercise.

Ingredients

½ organic lime with rind

1 organic cucumber with rind

1 large celery stalk

1 pound of Montmorency cherries, pitted

½ pound of fresh strawberries

1 green apple

Instructions

Place all the ingredients in a juicer and process. Serve immediately.

Tomato Juice

Yield: 1 serving

Lycopene is a compound found in tomatoes that not only enables faster tomato recovery, but also stabilizes blood sugar levels.

Ingredients

1 big handful of cilantro

1 tomato

1 organic lime with rind

1 organic lemon with rind

4 large carrots

Instructions

Place all the ingredients in a juicer and process to extract the juice. Serve immediately to enjoy the nutrients.

Athletes Juice

Yield: 1L

Ingredients

2-inch piece of ginger

8 kale leaves

1 large handful of parsley

3 celery stalks

4 carrots

3 apples

½ pineapple

Instructions

Peel the ginger and remove the rind from the pineapple.

Wash all the ingredients and process them in the juicer.

Serve and enjoy.

Race-day Juice

Yield: 1 serving

Ingredients

5 strawberries

½ lemon, pulped

2 beets, cut into quarters

Instructions

Put all your ingredients in a juice extractor and process until ready. Serve.

Immune Booster

Yield: 1 serving

Ingredients

10 grapes

1 orange, cut into small pieces

1 cucumber

3 kale leaves

Instructions

Put all ingredients in a juice extractor and process. Serve.

Post-race Recovery Juice

Yield: 1 serving

Ingredients

1 inch ginger root

1 cup of blueberries

2 cups of tart cherries, seeded.

Instructions

Put all ingredients in a juice extractor and process. Serve.

Orange and Broccoli Juice

Yield: 1 serving

Kiwifruit, orange, and broccoli are excellent sources of vitamin C necessary for the production of collagen. Collagen is the protein we need to maintain healthy skin, bones, and cartilage. This drink also provides iron, potassium, and vitamin A.

Ingredients

1 kiwifruit, peeled and chopped

1 cup (125g) of broccoli, chopped

1 large orange, peeled, seeded and chopped

Instructions

Process all the ingredients in a juicer and serve.

Pear and Peach Juice

Yield: 1 serving

These fruits have a low glycemic index giving a slow release of energy. It is, therefore, a good drink to have an hour before your workout or performance.

Ingredients

Filtered or spring water to taste

2 apricots, pitted and chopped

1 peach, unpeeled, pitted, and chopped

1 peer unpeeled, cored and chopped

Instructions

Process all the fruits in a juicer. Thin with a small amount of water if need be and enjoy.

Cucumber and Parsley Juice

Yield: 1 serving

Orange supplies vitamin C that helps your body utilize the iron in parsley. On the other hand, cucumber has a cooling effect and therefore useful after an event or workout. Spirulina is a "super food" high in many nutrients.

Ingredients

½ teaspoon of Spirulina powder

1 small cucumber

2 cups packed parsley spring with stems

1 large orange, peeled, seeded and chopped.

Instructions

Process the parsley, orange, and cucumber in a juicer and pour into a glass.

Stir in the Spirulina powder and serve.

Plum and Berry Juice

Yield: 1 serving

Go for the red-fleshed plum variety; they are higher in nutrients than the yellow-fleshed one. Plums are also rich in potassium electrolyte alongside vitamins A, C, and E. The berries provide vitamin C and bioflavonoids that strengthen arteries and veins.

Ingredients

3 large red-fleshed plums, pitted and chopped

1 cup (125g) of frozen strawberries, thawed

1 cup (125g) blackberries, frozen and thawed

Instructions

Process all the ingredients in a juicer and serve immediately.

Cantaloupe Juice

Yield: 1 serving

The vitamin C in pineapple and guava encourage the production of collagen, a protein that fosters healthy bones and cartilage. Cantaloupe and pineapple have a high water content that is good for rehydration. Pineapple is also rich in an enzyme called bromelain, which is an anti-inflammatory that promotes the repair of damaged tissues caused by sporting activities.

Ingredients

1 guava, unpeeled and cut into wedges

¼ pineapple, peeled, cored, and chopped

¼ cantaloupe, peeled, seeded and chopped

Instructions

Process all the ingredients in a juicer and serve.

Pineapple Juice

Yield: 2 serving

Fennel is a female reproductive tonic that could be very useful to menstrual problems in female athletes. This juice is not only refreshing; it is also rich in antioxidants, vitamins, and enzymes.

Ingredients

¼ fennel bulb, trimmed, cored, and chopped

1 lime, peeled, seeded, and chopped

¼ papaya, peeled, seeded, and chopped

½ pineapple, peeled, cored, and chopped

Instructions

Put all ingredients in a juicer and process; serve.

Melon and Grape Juice

Yield: 1 serving

Melons and lychees have a cooling effect on your body. This juice is therefore great to have after a workout. Grapes replenish energy first because they have a high glycemic index.

Ingredients

6 lychees, peeled and seeded

1 cup (125g) of grapes

½ small honeydew melon, peeled, seeded and chopped

Instructions

Process all the ingredients in a juicer.

Serve and enjoy.

Carrot and Ginger Juice

Yield: 1 serving

Ginger helps to stimulate circulation and aids in digestion. Carrot and orange contain the important antioxidants vitamins A and C. Ginseng gives a natural energy boost.

Ingredients

½ inch piece of fresh ginger

1 large orange, peeled, seeded and chopped

1 large carrot, chopped

½ cup (125ml) boiling water

1 ginseng tea bag

Instructions

Steep the ginseng tea bag in a cup of boiling water for 10 minutes then remove.

Refrigerate the tea for about 20 minutes.

Process the ginger, orange, and carrot in a juicer and pour into a cup.

Pour in the tea and stir to combine.

Serve and enjoy.

Papaya and Mango Juice

Yield: 1 serving

Because papaya and mango have a high glycemic index, this juice makes a great drink after an exercise or a performance; it quickly restores your lost energy.

Ingredients

1 mango, peeled, cut from pit and chopped

¼ papaya, peeled, seeded and chopped

1 ruby grapefruit, peeled, seeded, and chopped

Instructions

Process all the ingredients in a juicer and then serve.

Tomato and Cabbage Juice

Yield: 1 serving

Tomatoes, celery, and cabbage contain potassium and sodium electrolytes that are important for balancing the electrolytes in your body. Celery also has anti-inflammatory properties. This drink is, therefore, a good one to have after a workout.

Ingredients

2 celery stalks

1 cup (30g) of packed parsley springs with stems

1 1/3 cups (125 g) cabbage, chopped

1 ripe tomato, cut into wedges

Instructions

Process all the ingredients in a juicer and serve.

Chapter 5: Juice Recipes To Fight Inflammation

Inflammation of the muscles or in the body is never a good thing for athletes. These juice recipes will help you fight inflammation:

Green Juice

Yield: 1 serving

If you frequently feel low on energy, you may be anemic. The greens in this juice are a great source of iron. In addition, the ginger and lemon ensure maximum absorption and increase the speed of inflammation recovery.

Ingredients

1-inch ginger root

½ lemon

1 cucumber

A punch of parsley

2 green apples

8 leaves of kale

Instructions

Juice all the ingredients in your juicer, serve, and enjoy.

Green Pineapple Juice

Yield: 1 serving

The pineapple and ginger are effective anti-inflammatory foods that will help reduce inflammation and joint aches.

Ingredients

1-inch fresh ginger root

A few sprigs mint leaves

A big handful spinach

6 ribs of celery

1 cup of pineapple chunks

Instructions

Put all the ingredients in a juicer and process until ready. Serve and enjoy.

Ginger Beet Juice

Yield: 1 serving

If you routinely workout, then beetroot juice is a drink you should also routinely drink. Drinking it before your workout improves your stamina and endurance. Drinking it after help reduce inflammation.

Ingredients

1-inch ginger root

1 small lemon

5 beetroots

Instructions

Juice all the ingredients and enjoy.

Conclusion

Thank you again for downloading this book!

Make an effort of making your own energy drinks, as you will know the exact ingredients in them, and you will be consuming fresh nutritious ingredients full of the natural vitamins and minerals your body needs to operate at peak performance.

Finally, if you enjoyed this book, would you be kind enough to leave a review for this book on Amazon?

Click here to leave a review for this book on Amazon!

If you have received value from this ebook I recommended to read my other ebook you can find it here

https://www.amazon.com/dp/B06Y4C2TDB

Thank you and good luck!

5 Easy Juicing Recipes

How to Boost Your Energy, And Help Your Body
To Recover Faster

Introduction

I would like to thank you for downloading the book, *"5 Juicing Recipes How To Boost Your Energy, And Help Your Body To Recover Faster."*

Juicing has been around for quite some time and for good reason. Juicing ensures that the insoluble fiber is removed; leaving you with a juice that contains a high concentration of vitamins, enzymes, and minerals that can be quickly digested and absorbed into your bloodstream. This is especially important to athletes or those engaged in increased physical activity.

As you know, your body uses calories or energy to undertake activities. The tougher the activity, the more energy your body expends. If you expend too much energy, your body will break down and it may take you a long time to build it back up. Athletes who don't take care of their bodies often find themselves having a hard time staying on top of their game. On the other hand, faster recovery allows your body to rejuvenate and prepare for the next workout.

If you want to boost your energy and recover faster, it would be just a matter of knowing what your body uses up and how you can quickly replace such properties in order to experience fast recovery and this is what this book will be all about. You will also learn a few juicing recipes that will ensure faster recovery.

Thanks again for downloading this book, I hope you enjoy it!

Essential Nutrients And Minerals For Faster Recovery

Before learning more about the juicing recipes that boost your energy and ensure a quick recovery, it is important to understand the essential nutrients that your body needs for faster recovery. These nutrients include:

Glucose: glucose is stored in your muscle cells as glycogen. Your muscles use it during high intensity exercises. During exercise, you can lose up to 70% glycogen.

Fatty acids: These are stored in muscle cells as triglycerides and they are used as a secondary fuel source during low intensity workouts. As with glucose, your body can lose up to 70% triglycerides after a workout.

Amino acids: Amino acids provide the other source of fuel. Unlike glycogen and triglycerides, they are not stored inside the muscle cells; rather they are the storage tank itself or the muscle protein as it were. Your body will first burn glucose and fatty acids breaking down your muscles for energy.

It is also good to note that although amino acids are the last energy resort; your body will still experience what is known as muscle microtrauma. This is because of repeated muscle contractions. You have to repair your body as soon as you finish your workout to keep it in good shape.

After your workout, your body will be in dire need of energy. In fact, your cells will be very 'hungry' 2-3 hours after your workout. It is important to feed them before this window closes, as this is when the enzymes needed for glycogen synthesis, protein synthesis, and triglyceride synthesis are revved up and just waiting to do their job.

In the following chapters, we will look at the above three nutrients in detail that your body greatly needs for faster recovery.

1. Branched-Chain Amino Acids (BCAAS)

Most athletes say they had a 'good' workout after they've gone through a hard training session. This often means that they gave their workout everything they got and they are happy with the result. Unfortunately, hard training sessions also wreck havoc on your muscles. They destroy your muscle protein and cause you to have a longer recovery time and a higher starting point whenever you want to bounce back from the workout.

In order to prevent this, many are turning to BCAAS supplements. BOCAS are branched-chain amino acids that include leucine, valine, and isoleucine. They are the once that form the muscle protein building blocks. Thus, it is important to add some foods that contain BCAAS to your juices.

Foods that contain BOCAS include:

Milk

When you drink milk, you will get the needed BCAAs and thus, you will have no need for supplements. Milk also contains whey, a fast digesting protein that is very useful when it comes to muscle repair. This is why many agree that it is better to drink milk after a workout than to drink energy drinks.

Another good thing about milk is that you can take it with no preparation and you can also make protein shakes and add in whatever ingredients you deem necessary for energy and recovery.

Many athletes drink chocolate milk instead of consuming sports drink as this is said to provide better results when it comes to recovery.

Whey

Most bodybuilders are quite familiar with whey protein. This high quality protein has been used for years to promote muscle growth. Whey contains leucine, which is one of the BCAAs amino acids. This amino acid is very effective when it comes to preventing muscle loss. It also promotes improved strength. Another important thing whey does is help reduce inflammation.

Remember that any strain you put on your muscles contributes to the 'wear and tear'. Thus, you should not wait to see the significant damage before doing something to aide in recovery. Ensure that foods containing BCAAs make a frequent appearance in your juicing regime.

Carbohydrates

Your body requires energy in order for it to be able to carry out its various functions. Most of this energy comes from carbohydrates. When you increase your physical activity, you burn more energy. If you consume more carbohydrates than your body needs, your body ends up storing those excess carbohydrates in the form of fat. This is why those who don't engage in exercise and yet eat high-carb foods put on weight.

When you consume carbs, your body has a constant supply of blood glucose, which it uses to carry out its functions. Glucose is stored in your liver and skeletal muscles as glycogen. This is to ensure that your body keeps functioning even when you are engaged in strenuous exercise.

When you exercise or increase the intensity of your workouts, your body starts using the stored glycogen. This means that by the time you finish your workout, you will need to replenish your glycogen stores. You can do this by ensuring that your juices have adequate carbohydrates.

Below are fruits and vegetables high in carbohydrates that you should include in your juices:

Oranges

Oranges are not often associated with carbohydrates. In fact, the first thing that may come to mind when someone mentions the word oranges is that they are a good source of vitamins. But they are also a good source of carbohydrates. Juicing one medium orange (navel orange) can give you about 17.56grams of carbohydrates. Other oranges such as California Valencia orange can give you about 14.39grams per medium orange. Oranges give you fresh tasty juice that mixes well with other fruits and vegetables. Before juicing oranges, ensure that they don't contain any seeds in them. You can remove the peel and slice the orange in quarters before juicing.

Carrots

Carrots are not just good for the eyes. They are also good for your energy levels. A medium carrot (raw) will give you about 5.84 carbs. Select healthy and firm carrots that don't have 'soft' spots. Wash them well and remove any blemishes. You don't have to peel your carrots before juicing them. Just cut off the edges and they are ready to go.

Cherries

A cup of cherries can also provide you with needed carbohydrates. Sweet cherries have about 22grams of carbs while sour cherries have about 13grams of carbs. Cherries also add flavor to your juices and make them more palatable.

Milk

Milk contains lactose, a sugar that replenishes your energy stores after you've finished your workout. If your goal is to gain more body mass, you would be better of drinking whole milk. This is because whole milk has protein, which has ultimately proved better for gaining body mass than fat-free milk.

It is good to remember that if you are involved in strenuous activities, you need more carbohydrates; thus, you shouldn't be afraid of consuming more carbs especially when you want to engage in a strenuous workout.

2.Antioxidants

Antioxidants play a very important role in your body. They help prevent free radicals from messing up with your cellular structures and causing a cellular breakdown. Training often results in more free radicals being produced. Since these free radicals do not have electrons to be attached to, they go ahead to 'steal' electrons from other cells and this can lead to disastrous effects as it messes up perfectly good cells.

The work of antioxidants is to 'volunteer' their own electrons as it were so that free radicals can bond with them and become stable hence eliminating the need to steal other cells' electrons. Antioxidants work to neutralize free radicals and this, in turn, helps your muscle recovery and prevents cellular breakdown.

Foods that contain antioxidants include:

Apples

Apples contain vitamins and minerals that are useful in helping your body to recover. Apples have ascorbic acid (Vitamin C), a common antioxidant that plays many roles in the human body including fighting free radicals and helping your body to fight disease.

Apples also contain quercetin. This antioxidant has anti-inflammatory properties that can soothe sore muscles. Apples also have catechins, a natural antioxidant that helps improve both brain and muscle function.

What is great is that apples go well with other fruits when juiced and make green juices more palatable.

Strawberries

Strawberries are often added to milkshakes, smoothies, and juices and for good reason. They are rich in vitamins and minerals. For example, strawberries contain Vitamin C, one of the most powerful antioxidants. Vitamin C helps your body to fight against infectious agents. It also does the admirable job of countering inflammation and scavenging free radicals.

Strawberries also contain two powerful antioxidants. These are ellagitannins and ellagic acid. Not only do such antioxidants fight bacteria but they are also said to prevent cancer. They also help reduce inflammation and this is important if you work out frequently. Strawberries also contain procyanidins, antioxidants that contribute to the various health benefits of strawberries.

Other antioxidants present in strawberries such as lutein, zeaxanthin, and beta-carotene are useful in protecting the body against free radicals and ROS (reactive oxygen species).

When buying strawberries, you should choose those that are ripe and without blemishes. Check to see for signs of damage. The fruits should not 'leak' their juices as this shows they are already past their due date.

Cherries

One of the first things you notice about cherries is that they are pigment rich fruits. This is a good thing because their pigment is really anthocyanin glycosides. These polyphenolic flavonoid compounds give cherries their rich color. Another great thing about the anthocyanins is that they contain powerful antioxidant properties. They have anti-inflammatory properties and are quite effective especially for those suffering from chronic pain including fibromyalgia and sports injuries.

Another antioxidant present in cherries is melatonin. This antioxidant is said to cross the blood-brain barrier and cause a soothing effect to brain neurons. It also helps when it comes to regulating sleep cycles. Cherries also contain polyphenolic antioxidants. These include lutein, beta-carotene, and zeaxanthin. These antioxidants act to prevent free radicals from causing havoc to other cells.

Celery

Celery makes an appearance in many diets. You can eat it as a snack or add it to your juice. One thing that makes celery so important is that it is rich in antioxidants. Celery contains phytonutrients such as flavonols, phytosterols, phenolic acids, furanocoumarins, dihydrostilbenoids, and flavones. The flavonoids antioxidants include lutein, beta-carotene, and zeaxanthin. These antioxidants are great for boosting the immune system and dealing with free radicals. You can use celery seeds, celery leaves as well as the stem. However, many juice recipes often use the stem part only.

Turmeric

Turmeric is often used to spice up food but it can also be added to juices. Turmeric contains curcumin, a substance credited with adding its primary pigment and known for its antioxidant and anti-inflammatory properties. Turmeric also contains the famous powerful antioxidant; Vitamin C. Vitamin C protects the body from infectious agents and free radicals.

Cucumber

Cucumbers contain vitamin C and beta-carotene, which are known for their antioxidant and anti-inflammatory properties. Cucumbers also have various flavonoid antioxidants such as apigenin, quercetin, kaempferol, and lutein.

Cucumbers also inhibit the pro-inflammatory enzymes such as cyclo-oxygenase 2(COX-2). They also prevent overproduction of nitric acid thus reducing the likelihood of excessive inflammation.

Before juicing cucumbers, you should wash them thoroughly and remove blemishes. Don't peel the skin as it has minerals and phytochemicals. You can slice the cucumber to make juicing easier if you wish.

Peppermint

Peppermint has antioxidant and anti-inflammatory properties. Examples of antioxidants found in peppermint are Vitamin C and beta-carotene. Antioxidants help protect your body against oxidative stress that is brought about by free radicals. Peppermint also contains rosmarinic acid. This antioxidant neutralizes free radicals and helps to reduce inflammation.

Carrots

Carrots are rich in antioxidant such carotenes and vitamin C. Beta-carotene is an especially powerful antioxidant that is useful in protecting the body from harmful oxygen-derived free radicals. Vitamin C is also powerful and it guards against free radicals.

When purchasing carrots, you should select bright-colored roots that are firm. Avoid soft or flabby roots. Older carrots don't contain as much juice as the younger ones. Thus, avoid going for the bigger carrots in hopes of getting more juice.

Kale

Kale is listed among foods that are the most nutrient dense due to the abundance of nutrients it contains. One of the things that make it so useful in recovery is that it contains various antioxidants such as quercetin and kaempferol. These antioxidants have anti-inflammatory properties that can work to soothe your muscles after a tough workout.

Kale also contains Vitamin C and beta-carotene. These powerful antioxidants counteract oxidative damage by neutralizing free radicals. When your body undergoes oxidative stress, you will be susceptible to aging and diseases such as cancer. Thus, it is important to get rid of free radicals.

Oranges

Oranges are well liked around the world. They are also known as an excellent source of vitamin C. In fact, eating just one orange daily, you will meet your recommended vitamin C intake for the day. Oranges also contain antioxidants such as anthocyanins, hesperidin, lycopene, and beta-cryptoxanthin. These antioxidants play various roles in making your body healthier.

Lemon

Lemons are a source of vitamins and minerals. They contain antioxidants such as Vitamin C, hesperidin, Berio citrin, and diosmin. Vitamin C is useful in improving immune health and protecting the body from harmful free radicals. Hesperidin works to strengthen blood vessels and diosmin is useful in reducing inflammation. It also works to improve vascular muscle tone.

Before using lemons, remove the peel and the seeds. Lemons don't give you a lot of juice. You may have to use at least two when you want to prepare juice. The good thing about lemons is that they mix well with other fruits and vegetables. Thus, you can use them to add a different flavor to other juices.

A variety of antioxidants can be found in fruits and vegetables. Make it a point to juice such foods in order to get the needed boost to fight against free radicals. Remember that the more stable your cells are, the faster you will be on your road to recovery.

2. Creatine Monohydrate

Creatine is well known in the fitness industry. Many weightlifters take creatine supplements in order to increase their endurance and muscle mass. The good news is you don't have to take creatine as a supplement. Some foods you can juice will give you all you need. This is because your body naturally builds or synthesizes creatine from those foods. Non-vegetarians can get all the creatine they need from meat or fish. Vegetarians, on the other hand, need to juice foods that the body can use to synthesize creatine. These foods should contain certain amino acids the body will use to build creatine. These amino acids include:

- Arginine – sources of arginine include foods such as coconuts, peanuts, soybeans, oats, chickpeas, and walnuts.
- Glycine – sources of glycine include foods such as spirulina, soy protein isolate, sesame seeds, raw seaweed and raw watercress.
- Methionine – sources of methionine include foods such as oats, sunflower seeds, and Brazil nuts.

As you can imagine, some of these foods would be very difficult to juice. But for the sake of your recovery and energy, you can crush the nuts into powder before adding them to your juices. Coconut water can easily be added to your juices as it blends easily with other food ingredients. When choosing coconuts, you should go for ones that are healthy and undamaged. Remember, you will be using the water inside the coconut. If you select old, damaged coconuts, you may open them up only to find that there is no water inside.

Foods such as spinach, watercress, and seaweed can be chopped into pieces to make juicing easier. When buying spinach, avoid the ones that are wilted and instead select healthy leafy green vegetables.

And of course, soy protein isolate can be added to your juices to provide you with that needed boost and to aide muscle recovery.

3. Electrolytes

When you exercise, you sweat. Your body loses not only water but also electrolytes. When you don't have electrolytes, you can start exhibiting symptoms such as dizziness, nausea and muscle fatigue. This is why it is important to replenish electrolytes once you are through with your workouts.

Foods that contain electrolytes include:

Milk

Milk is known for its calcium. It is especially useful when it comes to improving bone health. Considering you engage in a lot of physical activity, it is advisable to focus greatly on your bone health. This is especially true for women who suffer the risk of osteoporosis.

Apart from containing calcium, milk also has electrolytes such as sodium and potassium. Sodium and potassium help retain fluids in the body. In other words, they are useful in helping your body rehydrate.

Turmeric

Turmeric has minerals such as calcium, potassium, magnesium, iron, copper, and zinc. Potassium is important as it helps to control heart rate and blood pressure. Turmeric is often found in powder form but you can also use the fresh root.

Cucumber

Cucumber is a great source of potassium. You can get up to 147mg of the electrolyte in 100g of cucumber. When selecting cucumbers, make sure they are firm and that they are either bright to dark green. Store the cucumbers in the refrigerator to avoid wilting.

Peppermint

Peppermint is one of the well-known herbs. It is often drunk as a tea and it can be used to flavor candy. Peppermint contains iron, magnesium, copper, calcium and potassium. These are useful elements when it comes to health and recovery.

Kale

Kale is a good source of calcium. Vegetarians are especially advised to include this food in their diet. Calcium, as you know, is good for bone health. Thus, if your intention is to keep your body in great shape through exercise or to engage infrequent workouts, it would make sense to ensure your bones are healthy and strong.

Kale also contains potassium and magnesium. Magnesium protects you from heart disease and potassium helps reduce blood pressure as well as reduces the risk of heart disease. Kale also contains carotenoid antioxidants such as lutein and zeaxanthin. These antioxidants are said to lower the risk of muscular degeneration.

Carrots

Carrots contain a healthy dose of minerals such as copper, manganese, calcium, phosphorus, and potassium. Manganese is useful in that it is used as a co-factor for superoxide dismutase, an antioxidant enzyme while calcium helps keep your bones healthy and potassium helps control heart rate and blood pressure.

Apples

There have been many speculations about apples throughout the years. But one saying that stands out has to do with eating an apple a day and keeping the doctor away. It is true that apples have many beneficial properties. They also contain electrolytes. Drinking apple juice will help replenish your electrolytes and get back your energy.

Coconut water

Coconut water is just the kind of beverage you need after you are done with exercise. It replenishes electrolytes and helps your body rehydrate. Coconut water contains sodium, calcium, potassium, and magnesium. When you drink coconut water, you won't have to rely on sports beverages for your electrolytes. The good thing about coconut water is that you can drink it as it is. You don't need to add sugar or other additives to make it more appetizing.

And of course, don't forget to drink water. Your body loses water faster than it does electrolytes. Drinking water helps revitalize the body and sets you on the right path to recovery.

Juicing Tips

Before we can juice, you will benefit greatly from some juicing tips below:

Chop the ingredients

You can make your work a little bit easier by chopping your ingredients before juicing them. This is especially true when it comes to fibrous greens such as celery and spinach. Sometimes when you juice such foods, your juicer may end up clogging up. Chopping the ingredients reduces the risk of this happening and makes the juicing process to be faster.

Observe cleanliness

Remember that you are going to drink the juice as it is after you finish juicing. You won't use heat to kill off unwanted organisms. Thus, you need to be very careful when preparing your juice. Thoroughly wash your hands and wash your fruits and vegetables. Remove any blemishes before juicing your ingredients. If you are going to chop the ingredients, ensure you do that on a clean cutting board.

Another thing you need to do is clean your juicer as soon as you finish juicing. If you leave it for later, you will struggle with removing dried pulp from the juicer. Keep your tools and your produce clean and you will have less to worry about.

Mix it up

It is good to experiment with different ingredients. Drinking the same thing especially if it is not to your taste can make you stop juicing altogether. In addition, too much of everything is bad and this includes vegetables such as kale and cabbage. Therefore, change up the ingredients and discover new ingredients.

Also, try to follow the 80/20 rule. That is, use 80percent of vegetables and 20percent of fruits to make your juices. This way, you can focus on building muscles instead of piling up on carbohydrates. If this is too hard, then start with 60% fruits and 40% vegetables. Once you are used to this ratio, you can change it to 50% fruits and 50% vegetables. Before you know it, your juices will be 80% vegetables and 20% fruits.

Keep it simple

You may be excited about juicing and trying out various different ingredients. While this is great, it can become quite overwhelming especially when you are starting out. Therefore, it is advisable to juice a few ingredients at a time. This will save time and juice a few ingredients will seem much simpler as compared to juicing 10 ingredients

Buy fresh ingredients

You should stick to buying fresh ingredients as much as possible. Fresh fruits and vegetables contain a healthy dose of vitamins and minerals. Canned food is often times enhanced with additives. Fruits normally contained added sugars to help them last longer. There is no need to consume added sugars when the fruits already have their own natural sugars. Also, try to buy organic as this reduces the chances of the foods being contaminated by pesticides.

Spice it

Who said that juices should only have vegetables and fruits? As you have read in previous chapters, certain herbs are quite effective in ensuring your recover faster. Thus, to make your juices taste better, you can add such herbs like ginger and turmeric.

Storage

Sometimes it is not possible to drink the juices immediately after you've prepared them. This means you need to store them. However, since the juices are mainly made up of fruits and vegetables, the chances of the juice going bad are high especially if the juice is not stored properly. Make sure you store the prepared juice in a glass jar and place in the refrigerator as soon as you finish juicing. Also, ensure that you drink the stored juice within 24 hours.

Make juicing a habit

Juicing should be a habit. It should be something you do regularly to make your body healthier. Keep in mind that although working out is good for your body, it does use up energy and you do end up sweating and losing electrolytes. It makes sense to replenish your resources so that you can keep up this good habit.

Also, buy a good juicer that will make your juicing enjoyable. However, at the end of the day, remember that your goal is to get the most out of your juices. Don't look at price alone, also consider what you will be getting out of your juicers.

Remember that juicing is good for you. It helps you recover faster and it boosts your energy levels. You can juice most vegetables and fruits. However, it would be advisable to include ingredients geared towards helping your body recover faster. Keep it fresh. Keep it clean and keep it organic if you can. Above all, have fun trying out the various recipes in the following chapter.

5 Juicing Recipes To Help Your Body Recover Faster

Restorative Cherry Juice

Servings: 1

Ingredients

½ organic lime (rind included)

1 organic cucumber (rind included)

1 large celery stalk

1 pound of Montmorency cherries (remove the pits)

1 green apple

½ pound of fresh strawberries

Directions

Wash the ingredients, remove pits, cut off undesirable parts, and place the ingredients in a juicer. Juice, serve, and enjoy.

Cucumber-coconut

Servings: 2

Ingredients

Dash turmeric

8 ounces coconut water

2 mint leaves

1 green apple

½ cucumber

½ cup honeydew

Directions

Juice the ingredients and serve.

Protein Power Juice

Servings: 1

Ingredients

1 yam (sweet potato)

1 handful of almonds

1 orange (peeled)

1 apple

Directions

Wash the ingredients and ensure you gently scrub the yam or sweet potato. Peel the orange and then process the ingredients in a juicer. Serve.

Blueberries shake

Servings: 1

Ingredients

1 small cup of blueberries

½ mango

500ml milk

Directions

Juice the berries and mango. Pour the juice into a glass, add the milk, stir and enjoy.

Blood Cleanser Juice

Servings: 1

2 sprigs parsley

2 radishes

½ apple

5 medium carrots

6 leaves of spinach

1-inch piece of ginger

Directions

Juice the ingredients, serve, and enjoy.

Conclusion

Thank you again for downloading this book!

I hope this book was able to help you to learn about juicing recipes to boost your energy and help your body recover faster. The next step is to start juicing and take juices instead of relying on energy drinks.

Finally, if you enjoyed this book, would you be kind enough to leave a review for this book on Amazon?

Click here to leave a review for this book on Amazon!

Thank you and good luck!

www.ingramcontent.com/pod-product-compliance
Lightning Source LLC
Chambersburg PA
CBHW071240220526
45468CB00002B/942